Living with a Black Dog

How to take care of someone with depression
while looking after yourself

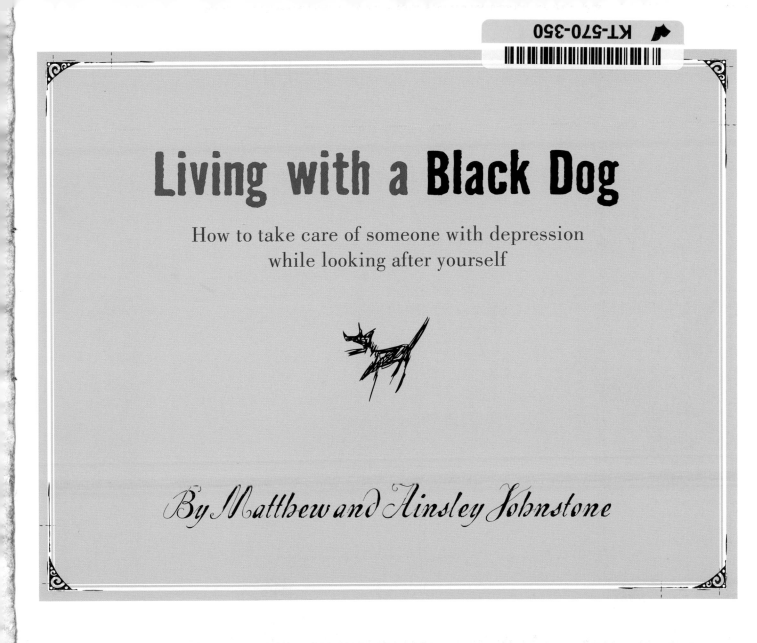

By Matthew and Ainsley Johnstone

Dedicated to 'man's best friend', the caregiver

Thank you

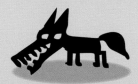

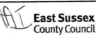

Living with a Black Dog

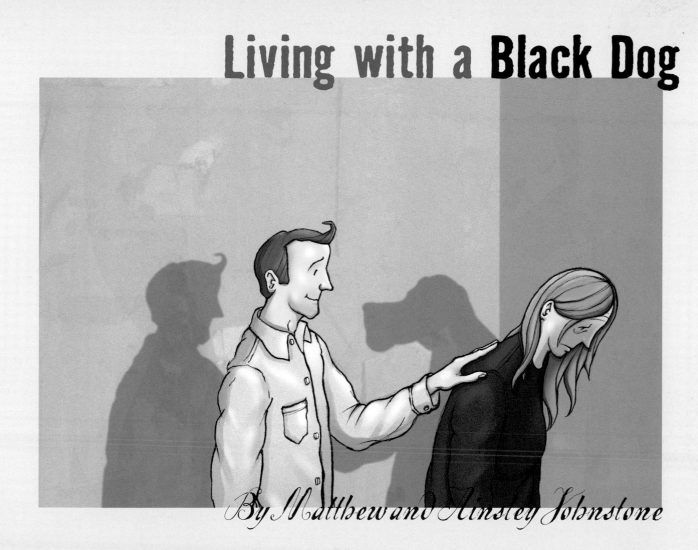

By Matthew and Ainsley Johnstone

ROBINSON

ROBINSON

First published in Australia in 2008 by Pan, an imprint of Pan Macmillan Australia Pty Limited
1 Market Street, Sydney

First published in the UK by Robinson, 2008

A CIP catalogue record for this book
is available from the British Library.

ISBN: 978-1-84529-743-5

Printed and bound in Italy by L.E.G.O. SpA

Robinson
An imprint of
Little, Brown Book Group
Carmelite House
50 Victoria Embankment
London EC4Y 0DZ

An Hachette UK Company
www.hachette.co.uk

www.littlebrown.co.uk

Important Note
This book is not intended as a substitute for medical advice or treatment. Any person with a condition requiring medical attention should consult a medical practitioner or suitable therapist.

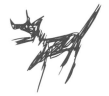

PRAISE FOR *I HAD A BLACK DOG* by Matthew Johnstone

'What a fascinating book. It is both instructive and accessible. I am sure it will have a universal appeal.'
Dr Rosemary Leonard, resident medical adviser for BBC1's *Breakfast*

'It's very accurate – I should know!' Ruby Wax

'Describing the hell of depression to other people, even those who really want to help, can be so daunting that sufferers find it impossible to reach out. Matthew Johnstone's cartoon book about confronting and ultimately befriending his own black dog cuts through the taboos in a simple, effective and touching way.'
Sarah Stacey, Health Editor, *YOU* magazine

'Truthful, touching and hopeful.' Dr James Le Fanu, medical columnist, *Daily Telegraph*

'His highly original mix of genres – autobiographical/self-help in picture-book format proved just what the doctor ordered.' Spectrum, *Sydney Morning Herald*

'This brilliant, disarming book about depression is quick to read, clever and poignant.'
Australian Financial Review

Foreword

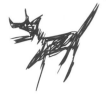

When Matthew initially said, 'I have depression', I really had no idea what that meant.
We were in love, the future looked bright, and I just thought we could face whatever it was together.

I had never dealt with depression and I certainly didn't know how it could and would affect me.

Which, in many ways, is exactly why we decided to create this book.

Caregivers live in the shadow of the Black Dog. As with any illness they take on the burdens, pick up the pieces and do all the worrying, often not knowing where to turn and what to do. Often they feel like they are walking on eggshells which can be exhausting, frustrating and upsetting.

However, the caregiver's role is a vital one. It can have an immeasurable impact on a loved one's recovery. Not only do they provide support, they are able to monitor the sufferer's healing process outside doctor visits. They also have a better understanding of the sufferer, their situation and circumstances.

Talking to people who shared a similar path to mine while researching this book made me realise the importance of sharing your experience with others. It's incredibly comforting to know you are not alone.

Recovery is all about acceptance and management by both the sufferer and the caregiver. It's something that Matthew and I have been able to do together through honesty, diligence, compassion and as much humour as possible.

It certainly put the old marital saying 'in sickness and in health' to the test but, at the same time, opened all our lines of communication and set us on the path of a deeper and more meaningful relationship.

We hope this book will shed some light into what your loved one's Black Dog looks like, and guide you both on the road to recovery. Depression is a treatable illness, not a life sentence. It does pass.

Ainsley Johnstone

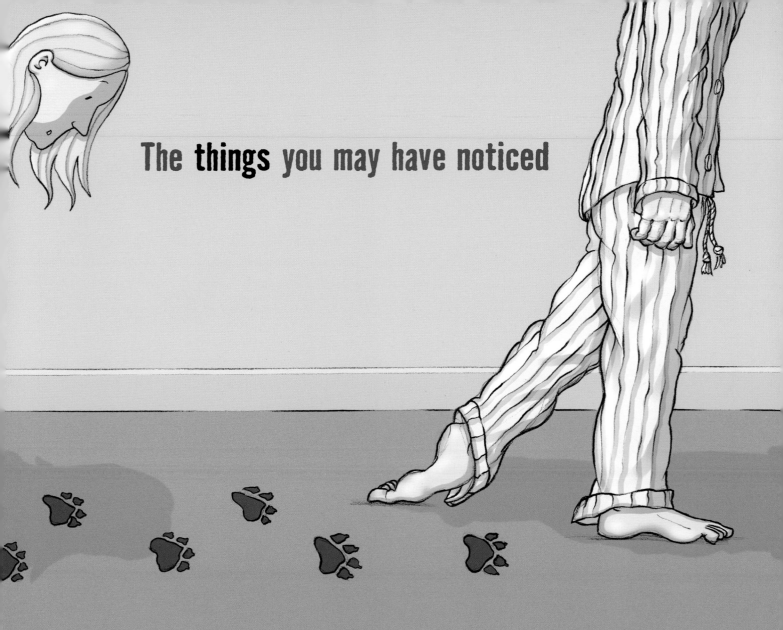

The things you may have noticed

You may have noticed they've lost the sparkle in their eyes.

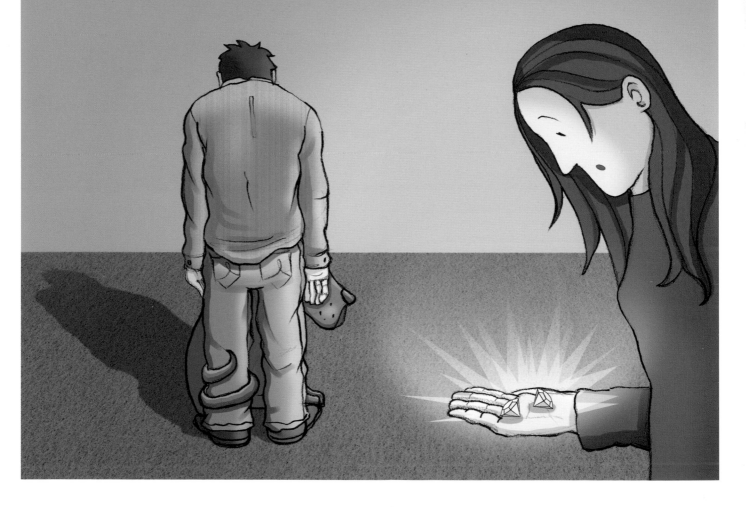

They may have an overwhelming
sense of tiredness which no amount
of sleep seems to cure.

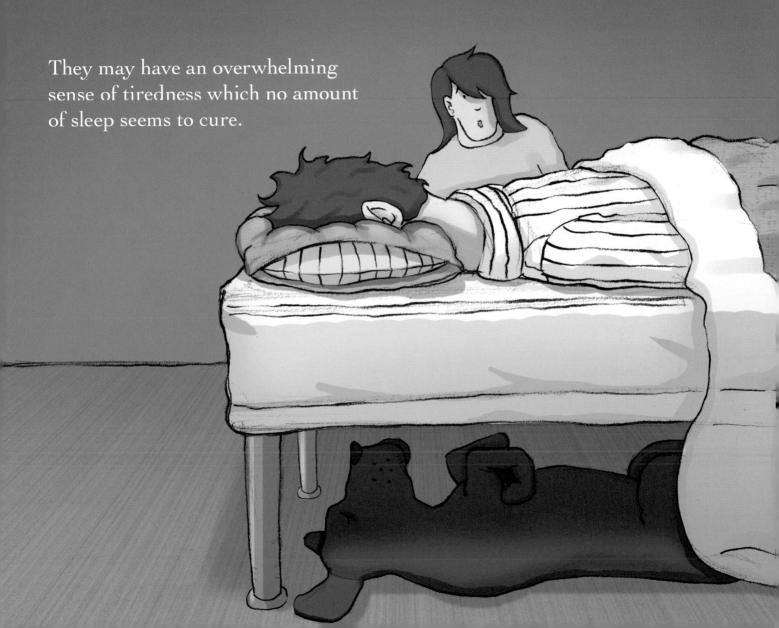

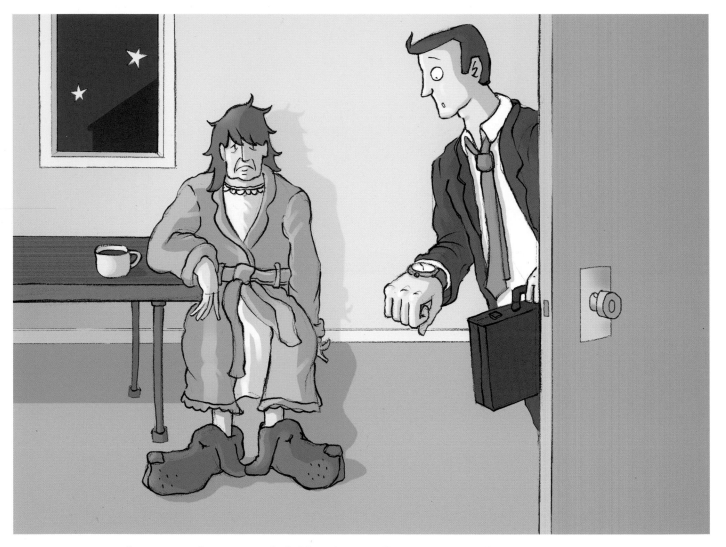

They may have real difficulty in firing-up and getting going.

A gradual slip in personal appearance,
hygiene and even memory is not uncommon.

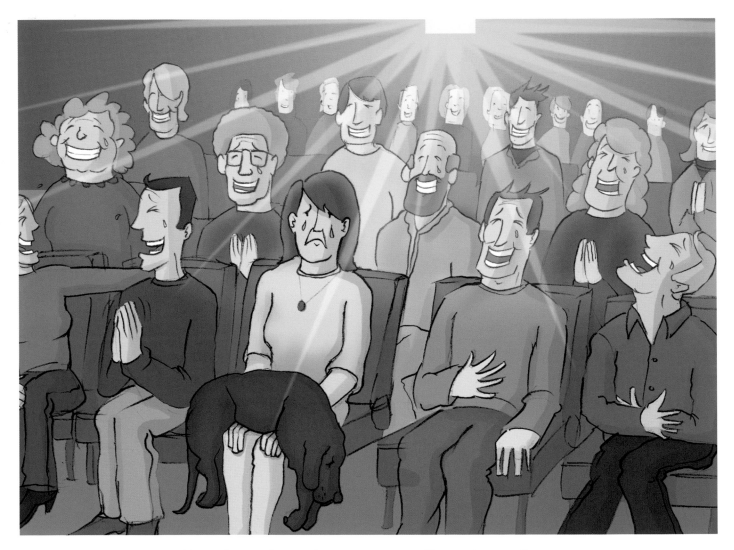

Laughter doesn't come as easily as it used to.

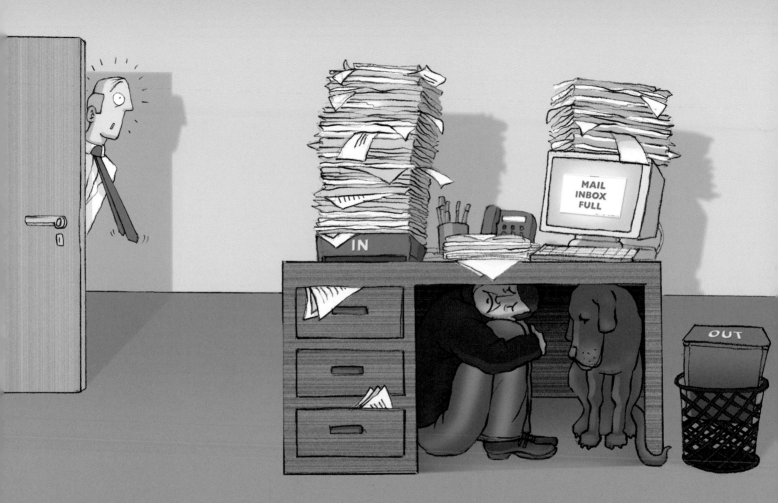

At work they may miss deadlines, make excuses for poor performance
and take more sick days due to 'other' ailments.

They may gradually withdraw from social events and other typically enjoyable activities.

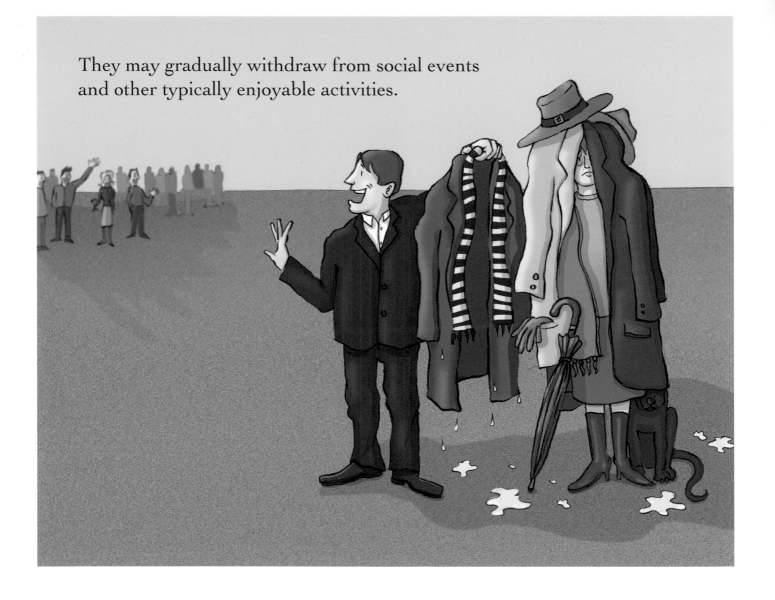

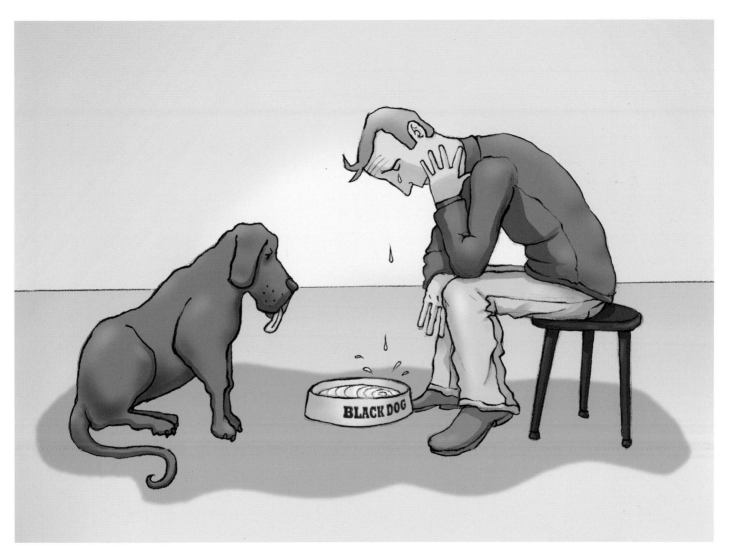

They may have become ultra-sensitive and cry more than usual.

Although exhausted, they may not
be able to relax or sit still.

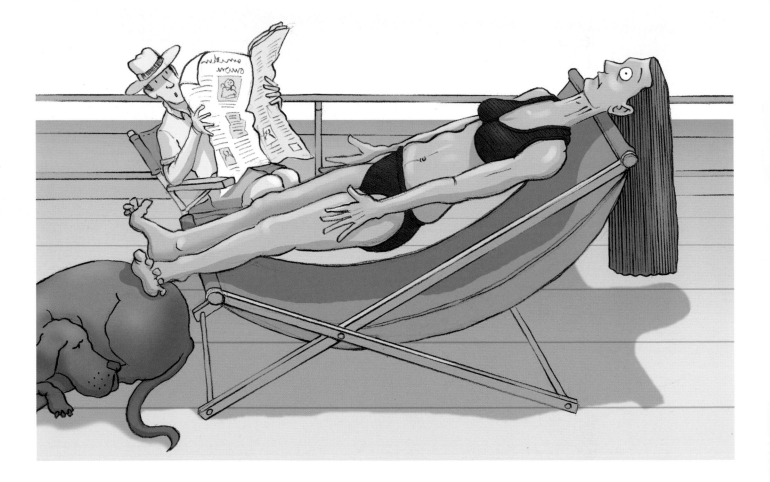

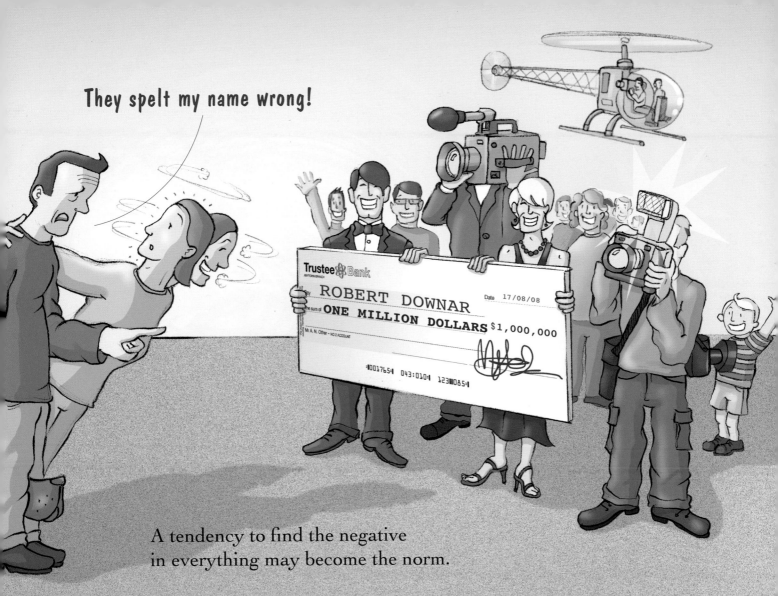

A tendency to find the negative
in everything may become the norm.

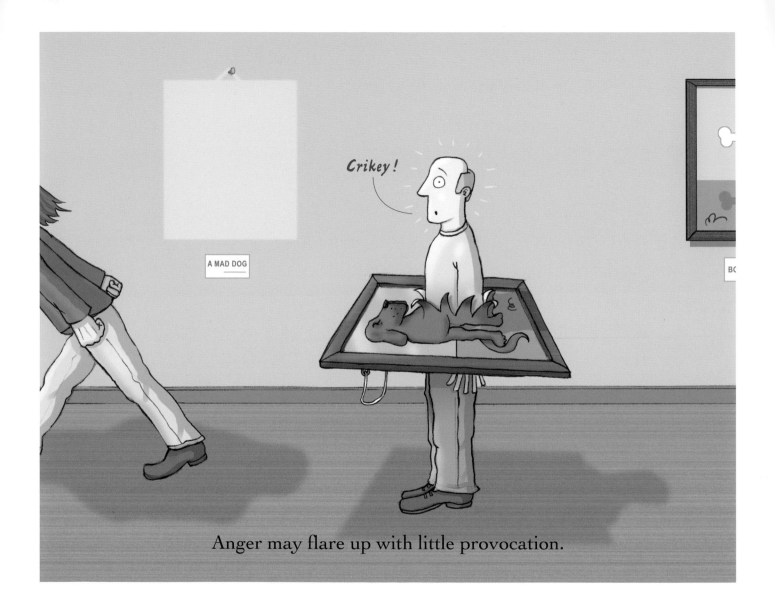

Anger may flare up with little provocation.

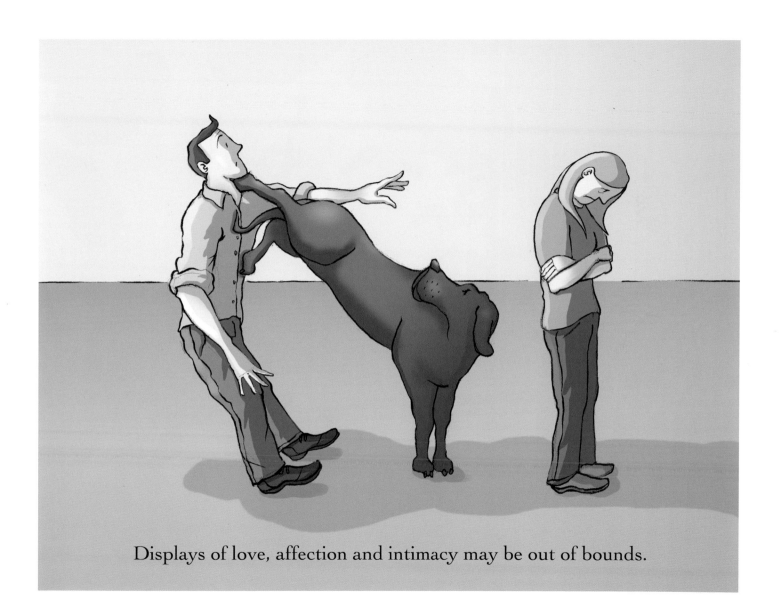

Displays of love, affection and intimacy may be out of bounds.

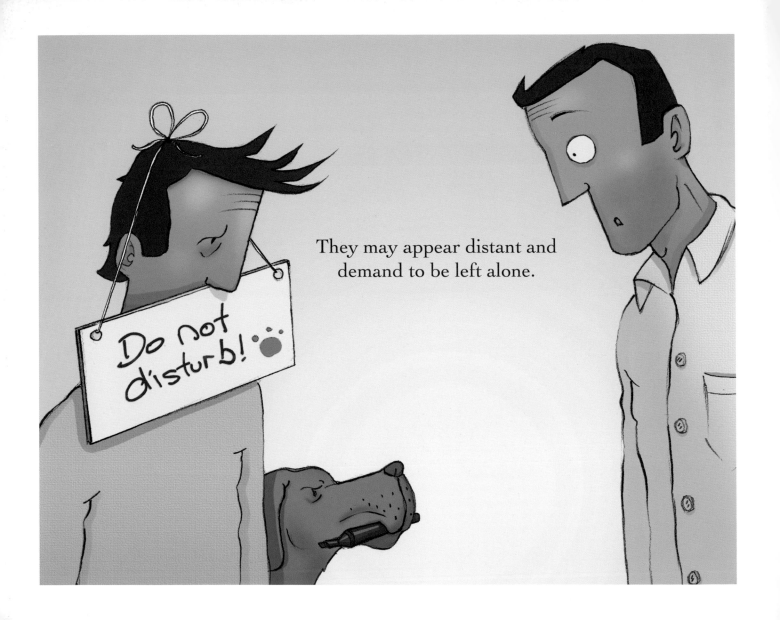

They may appear distant and
demand to be left alone.

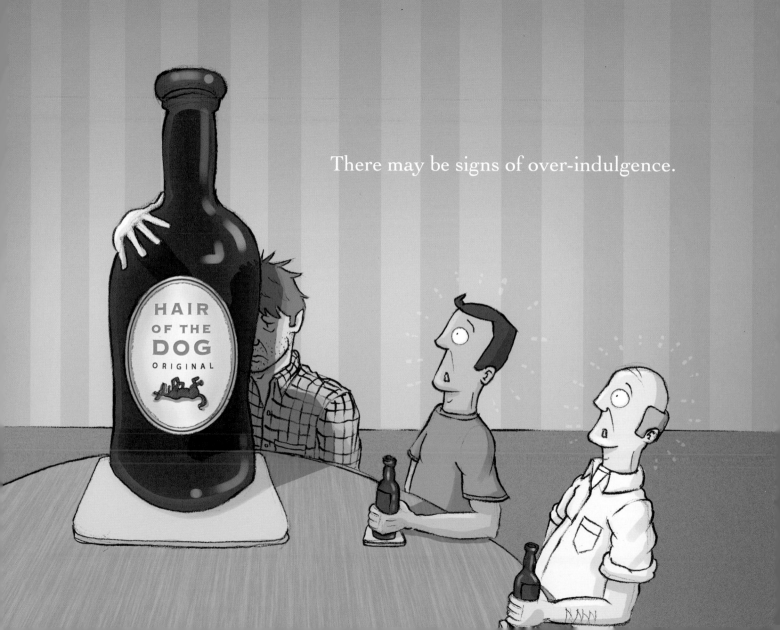

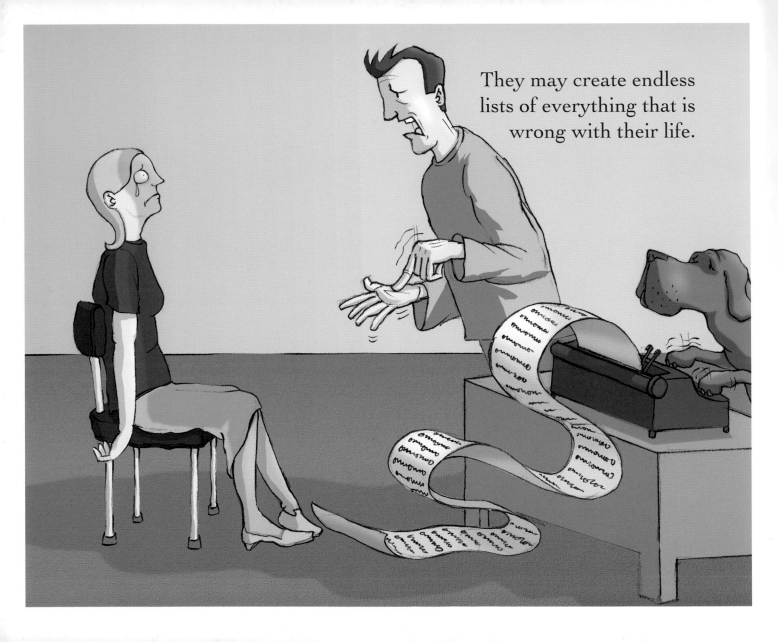

They may create endless lists of everything that is wrong with their life.

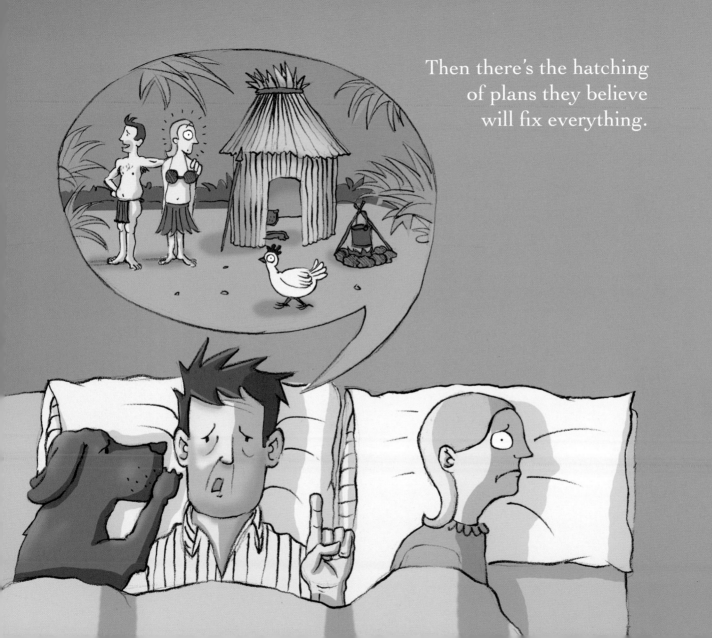

Then there's the hatching
of plans they believe
will fix everything.

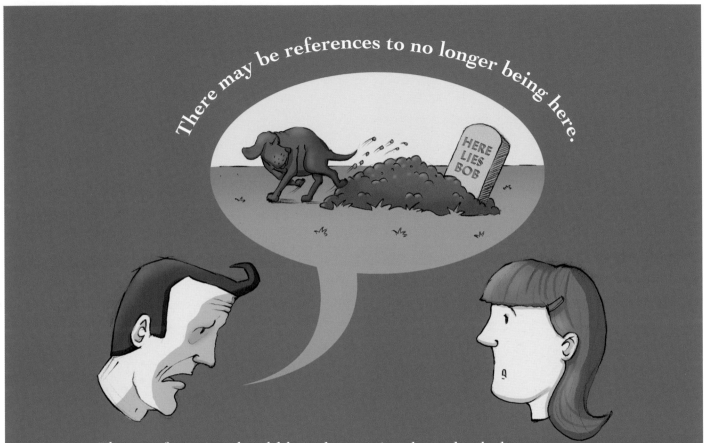

There may be references to no longer being here.

These references should be taken seriously and calmly.
Don't be afraid to talk about them. Ask them to clarify their
thoughts and, if concerned, call their doctor or a crisis support line.

What **not** to say or do

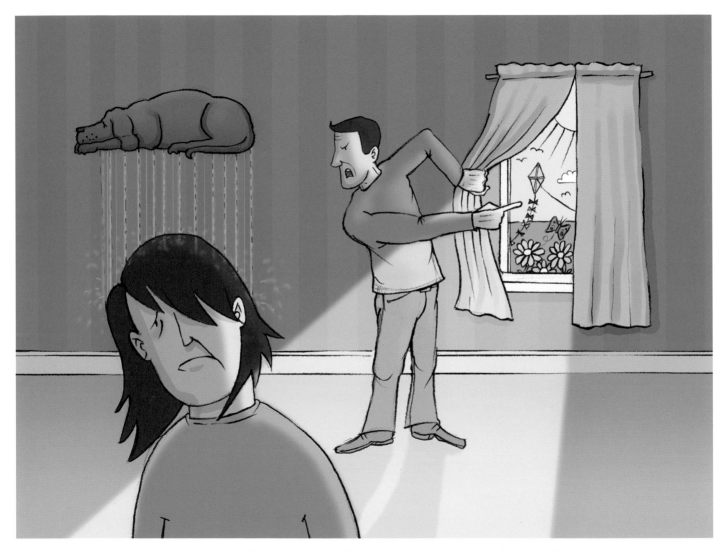

Pointing out lovely weather is annoying and pointless.

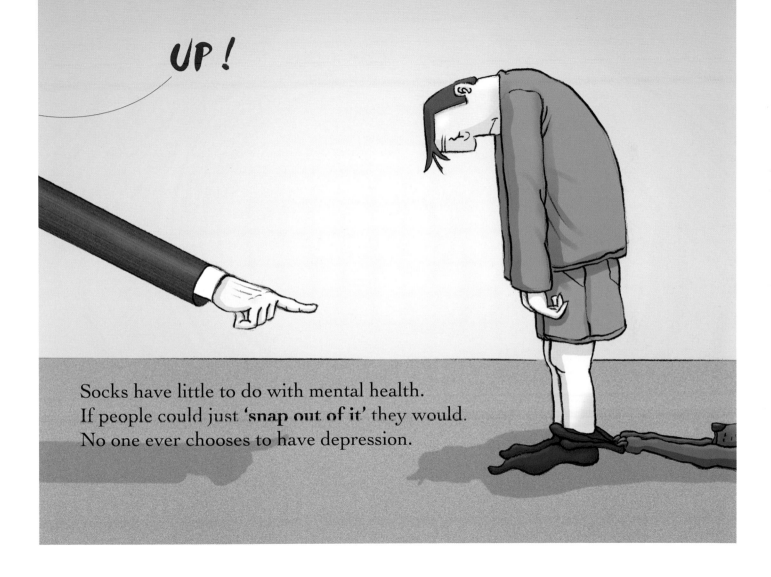

You may well be right when you say
'It's all in your head!',
but don't say it.

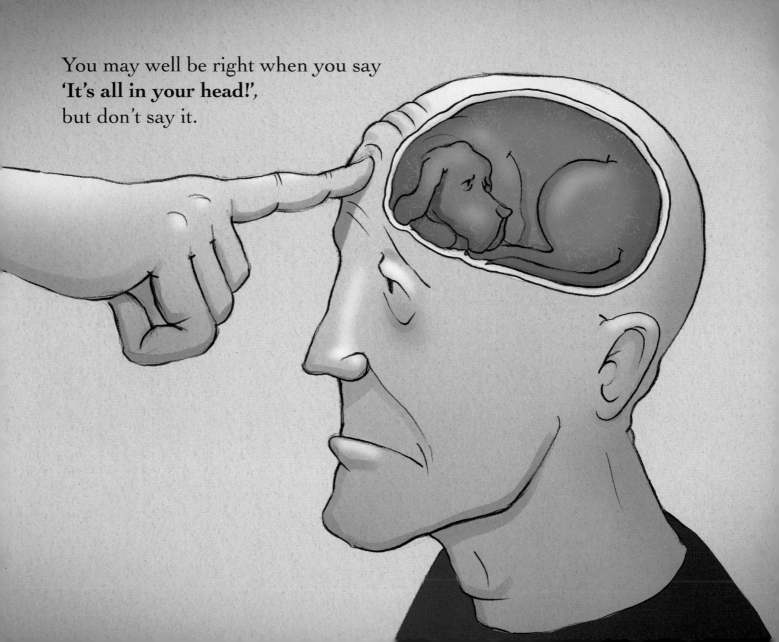

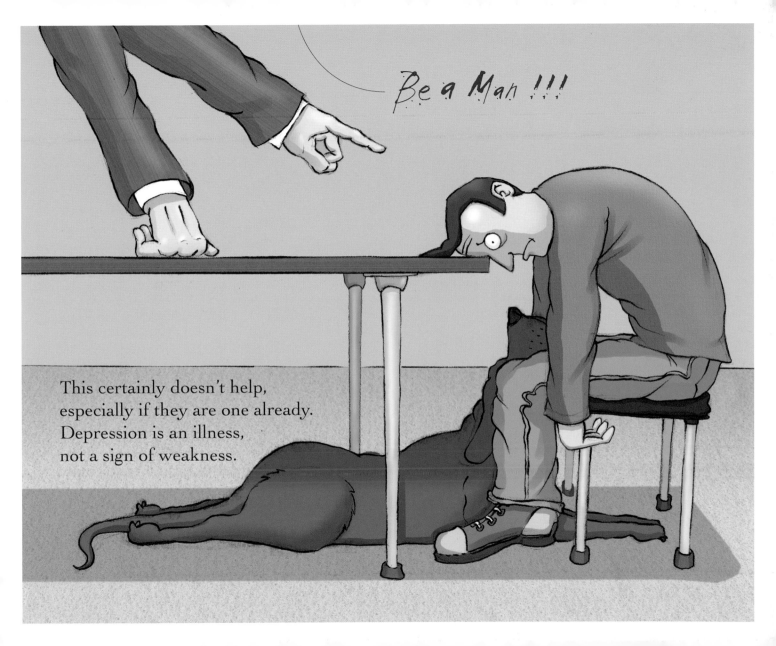

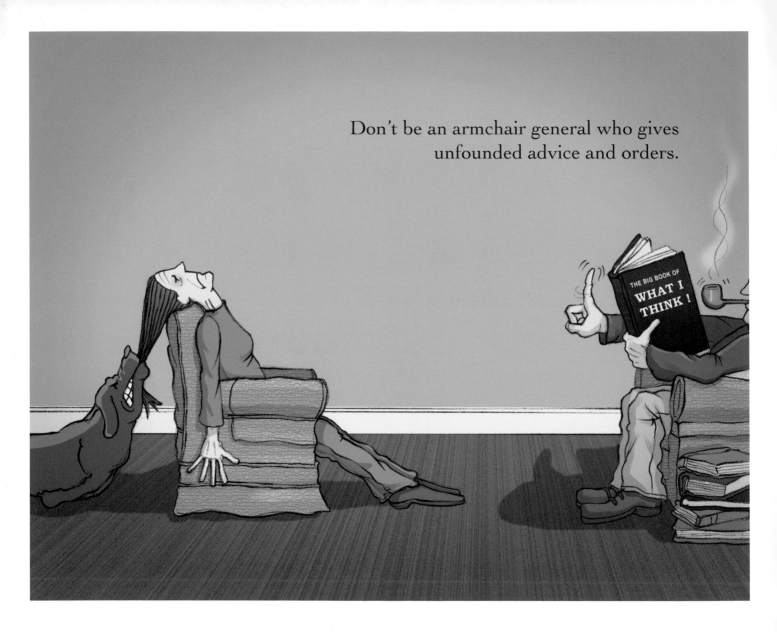

Being thoughtful and kind will never go amiss but don't try and jolly them along, it can often make them feel worse.

Never tell them they're **'just looking for attention'**;
it's demeaning and hurtful.

They're not looking for attention,
they are probably in need of it.

Don't point out that there are people in this world far worse off than them. It just adds to their feelings of guilt and hopelessness.

He just missed out on the Spiderman suit.

Don't push them into things they don't want to do and then make excuses for their behaviour. This only feeds the despair and keeps the denial alive.

Good things to say and do

Be sensitive about how you approach the subject;
a lot of people aren't used to talking
about their mental health or lack of it.

Crossing that line simply means you care.

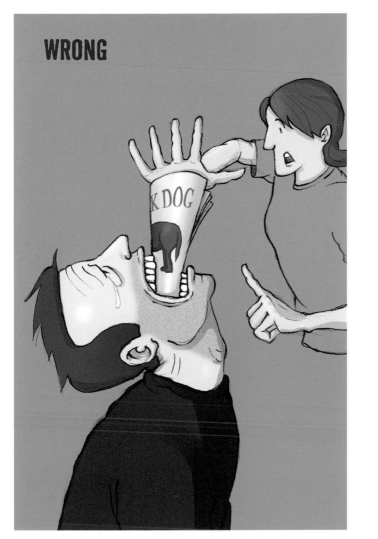

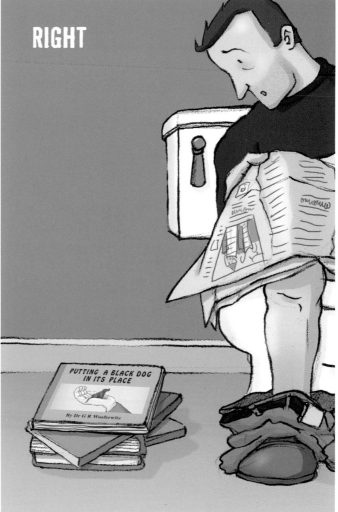

If you're going to share relevant information, be subtle in how you go about it.

Try not talking. **Just listen.** Really being there for someone without opinion or judgement is one of the best gifts you can ever give.

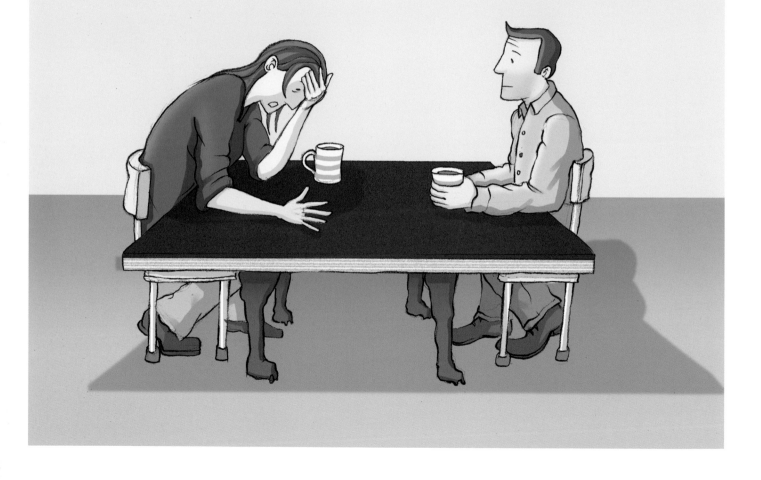

If receptive, encourage them to seek a professional opinion.
An offer to help find a good doctor, make an appointment
and even to go with them, can be hugely beneficial.

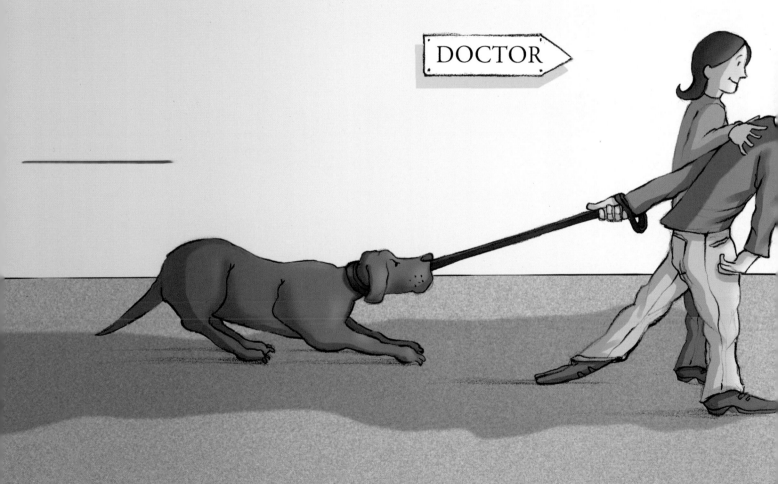

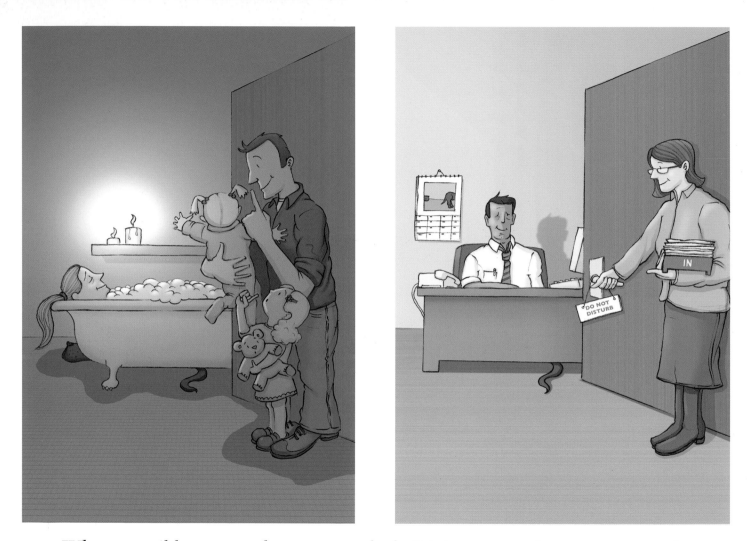

Where possible, try to take up some slack. It's important, however, not to do everything for them. A degree of routine is vital for self-esteem and self-respect.

Encourage any form of regular exercise.
Fitness robs the Dog of its power.

If you're genuinely worried about someone, organise a group of close friends or family members to make some sort of contact each day.
It can be to help out, have a coffee or simply to say hello.

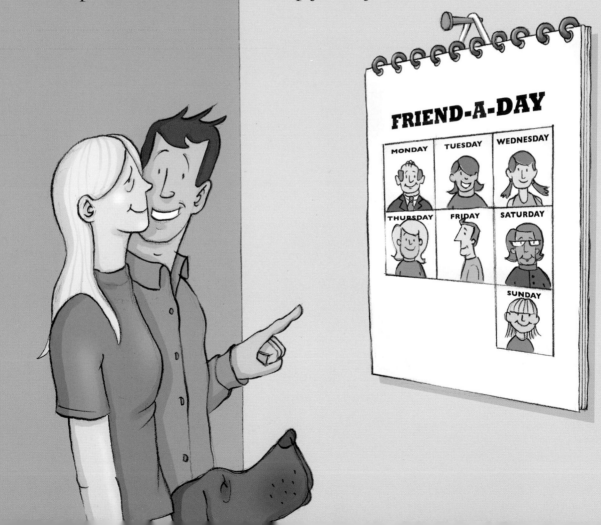

Help them develop a strategy to simplify
their life both at home and at work.
Stress is one of the biggest drivers
of depression. **Less stress, less dog.**

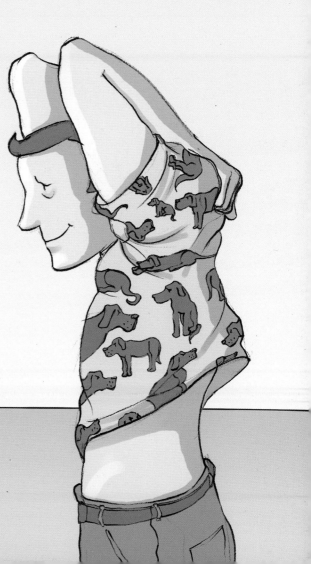

Make them a **'Ditch the Dog'** box. Encourage them to fill it with favourite photographs, letters – anything that reminds them of what's good in their life.

Include a **'White Dog Journal'**; here they can acknowledge progress, record the things they are grateful for and set do-able goals.

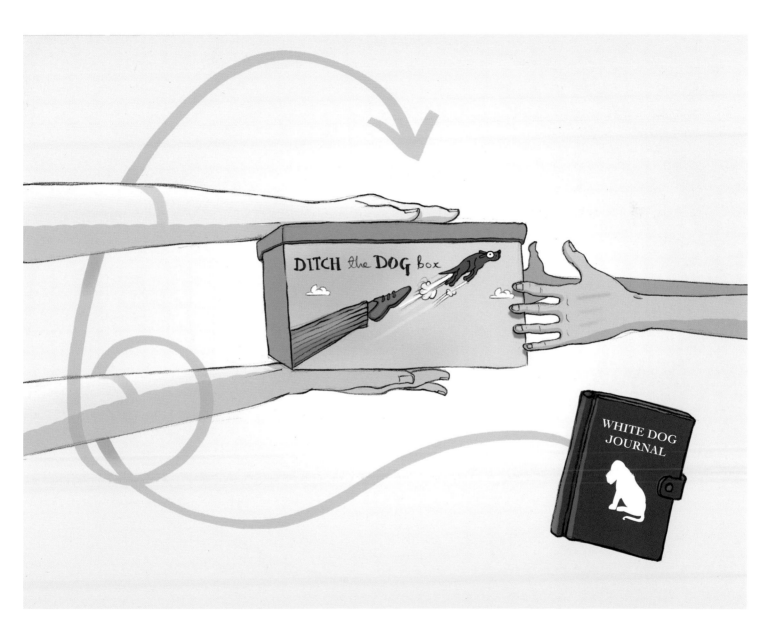

Embracing the Black Dog

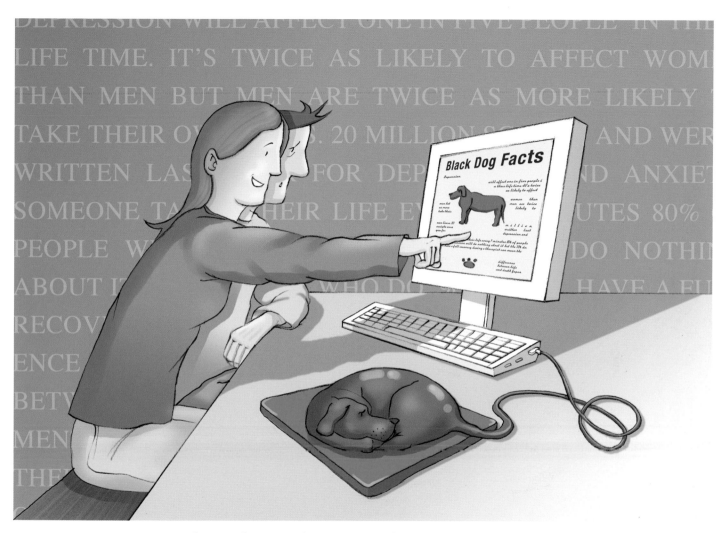

Learn about the condition together; knowledge is power
and validation is a great healer.

Take a united front and get
M.A.D at the Black Dog.

M is for **Management**. Manage the condition by taking responsibility for lifestyle choices, and stress levels.
Manage these and you are more able to manage the Dog.

A is for **Acceptance**. Accept that depression is an illness and like most illnesses it can be cured. Accept help where and when it's offered.

D is for **Discipline**. The discipline to see the doctor, to take the medication if required, to communicate clearly, to exercise regularly, to rest well and to eat well. Have the discipline to **discipline** the Dog on a daily basis.

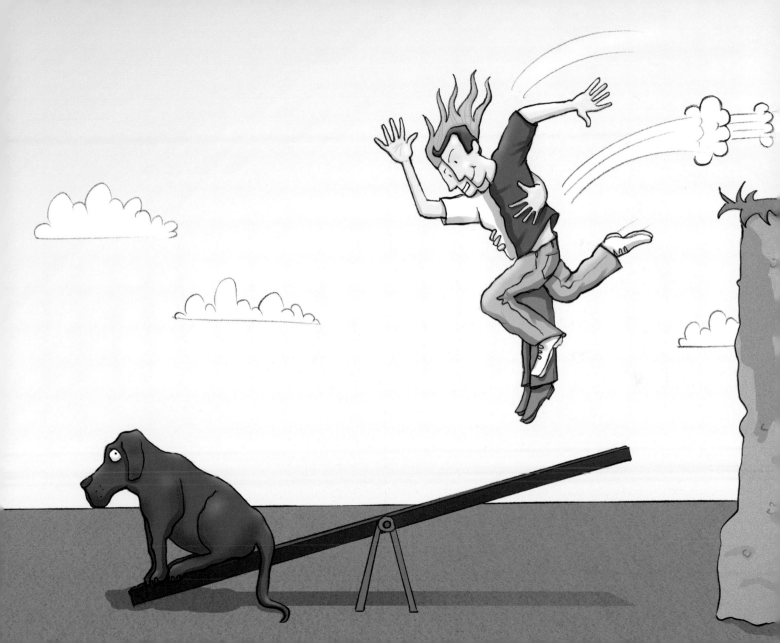

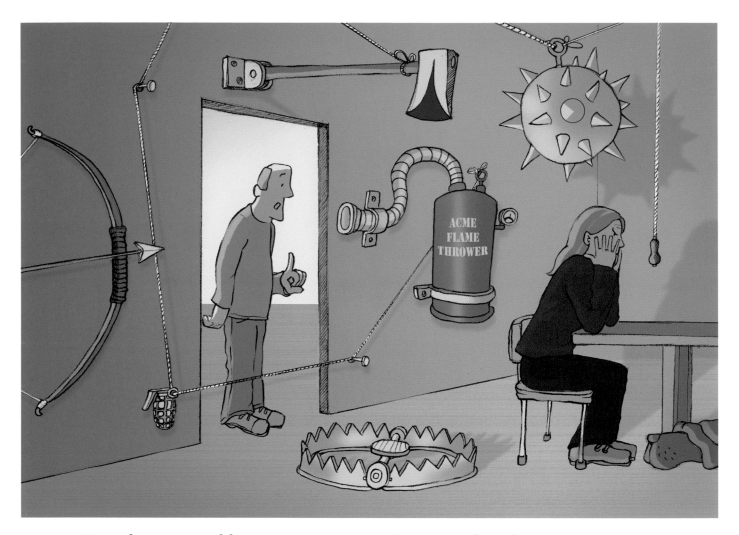

Together, try and learn to recognise triggers and early warning signs.
Also know when to give each other a bit of space.

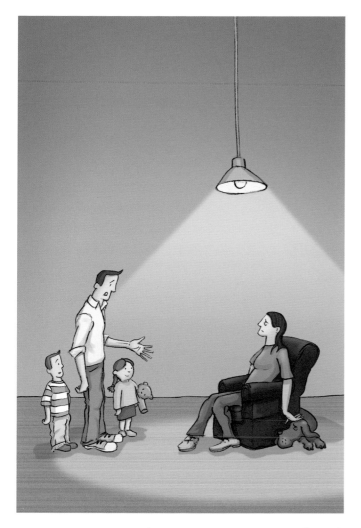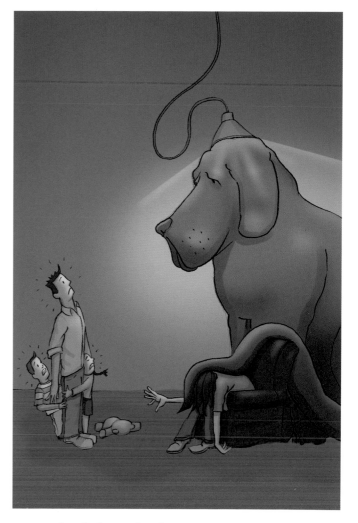

Agree to a course of action to get rid of the Black Dog.
An ignored Dog can become a big problem.

If they're old enough, inform children about what's going on. They need to know that the Black Dog isn't here to stay. Children often think it's their fault; reassure them that it's not.

As a caregiver, compassion, empathy and understanding are vital, but recognise that you alone don't have the power to rescue your loved one.

Professional help is often what's needed.

A big obstacle for seeking professional help is the cost.
Help them realise that the cost of not getting the right help can be
considerably higher; it can cost marriages, friendships, jobs and even life itself.

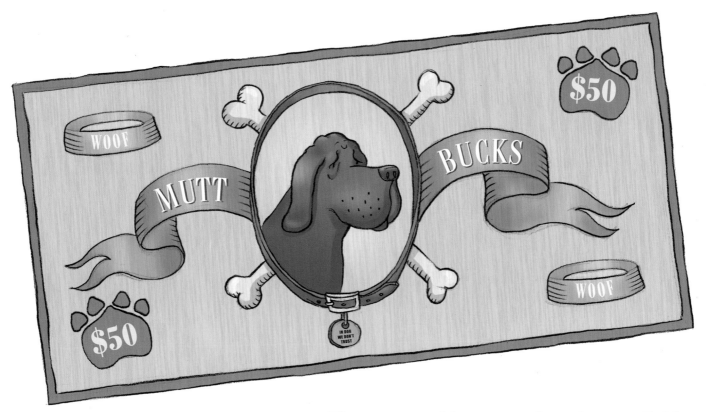

There are a wide range of services available;
as a starting point, see the list at the back of this book.

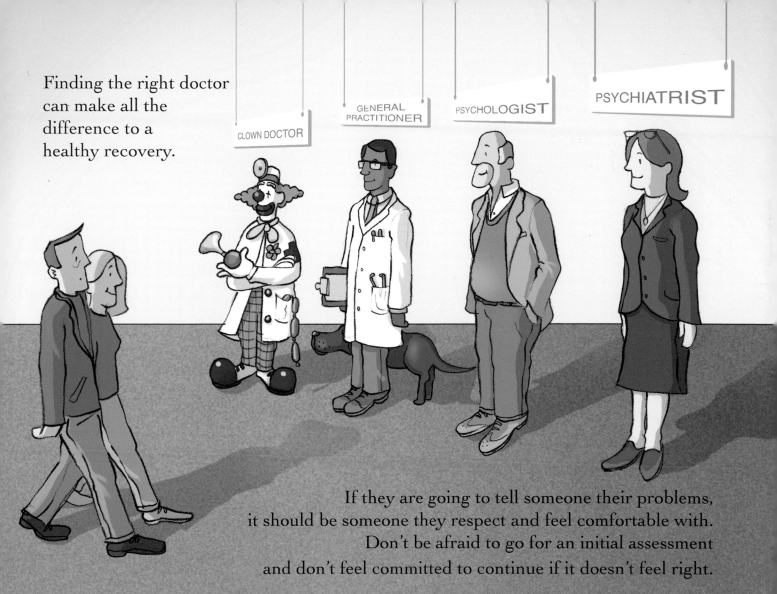

Finding the right doctor can make all the difference to a healthy recovery.

CLOWN DOCTOR

GENERAL PRACTITIONER

PSYCHOLOGIST

PSYCHIATRIST

If they are going to tell someone their problems,
it should be someone they respect and feel comfortable with.
Don't be afraid to go for an initial assessment
and don't feel committed to continue if it doesn't feel right.

There is a glossary of mental health practitioners at the back of the book.

Depression can be a chemical imbalance in the brain which is why it can sometimes make sense to take chemicals to rectify it. Antidepressants may be vital for some but they are not for everyone.

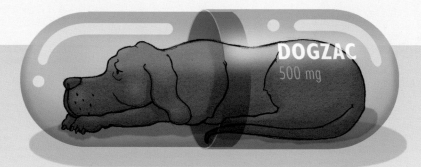

There is also a wide range of natural remedies that can help relieve symptoms. Do lots of research, know the facts and ask your doctor plenty of questions.

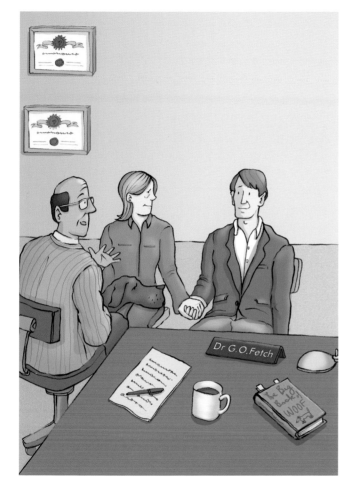

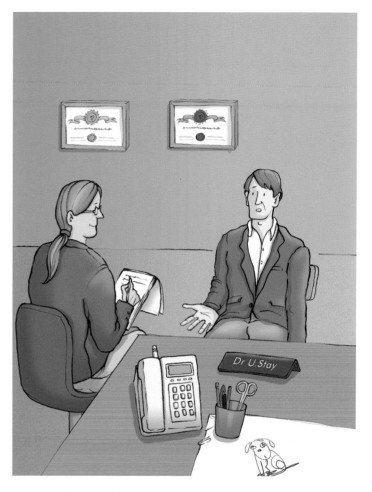

Seeing their doctor can help you understand what they might be going through. You can also get some insight on how to navigate your relationship during this period.

'Carer fatigue' is not uncommon, and it can pay to see your own doctor. It's a safe haven to share your own story and, most importantly, get support.

SOME SIMPLE RULES of ENGAGEMENT and AGREEMENT

1) Agree that there is a Black Dog in your midst and that things may have to change temporarily.

2) Agree that no one can help them until they fully commit to helping themselves.

3) Agree to be gentle and respectful with one another during this time.

4) Agree that ill-tempered behaviour is not necessary and won't be tolerated.

5) Agree to 'check in' with each other on a regular basis.

6) Agree to communicate honestly and openly.

7) Agree to the course of action set by their doctor and to review progress regularly.

8) Agree on a fallback plan (like the one at the back of this book).

Sign here ....   *Sign here* ....

Self-preservation for the Caregiver

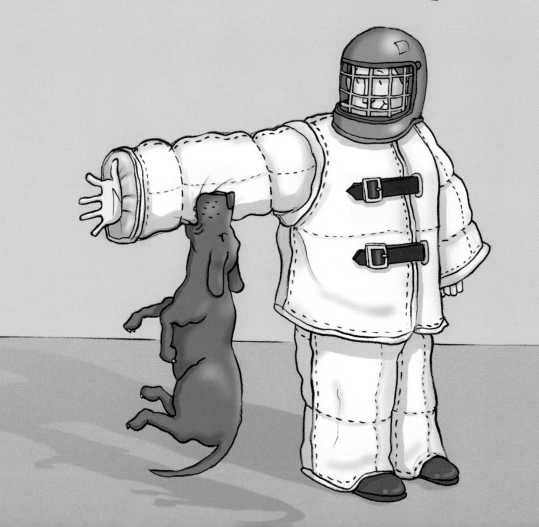

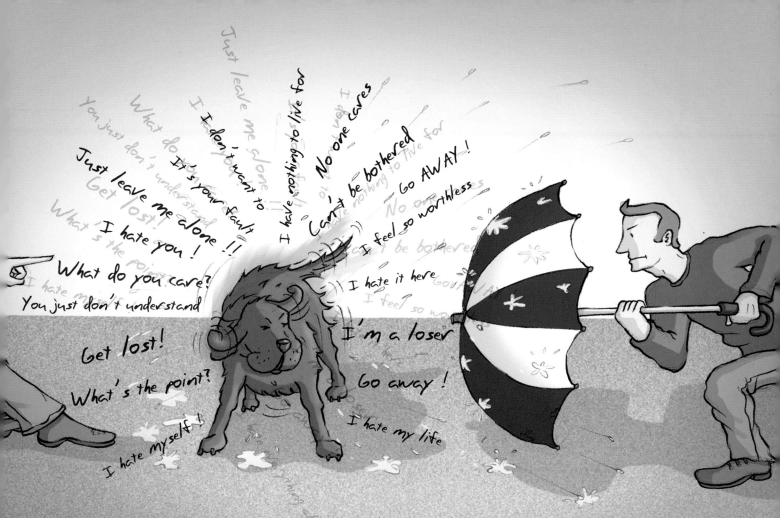

It can be difficult not to take anger, criticism, negativity, and apathy personally.
It's important not to buy into it; accept that
it's the depression barking, not the person you care for.

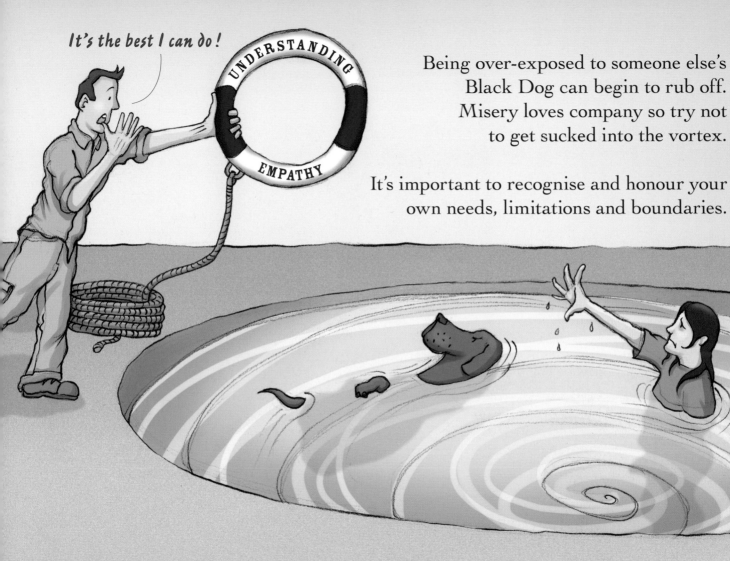

Write down ten things you love and know to be true about that person. Share it with them, keep it close by and put a copy in their 'Ditch the Dog' box.

Difficult situations are better dealt with when
you are calm and in the moment.
Yoga and meditation are great tools for
achieving calmness and control
(this also applies to the sufferer, so try to
encourage them to join you).

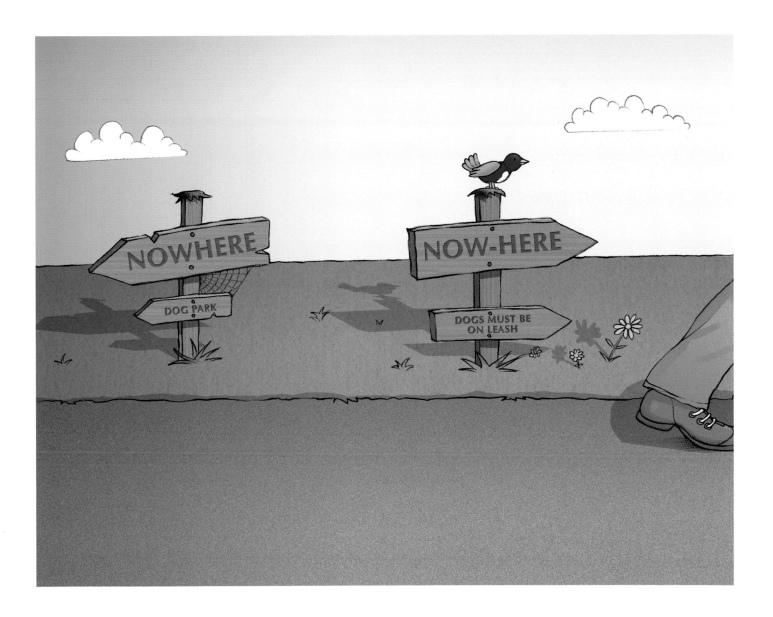

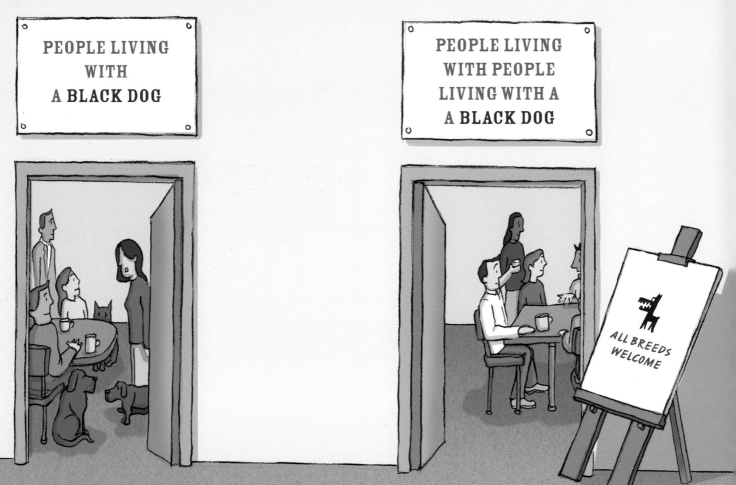

PEOPLE LIVING
WITH
A BLACK DOG

PEOPLE LIVING
WITH PEOPLE
LIVING WITH A
A BLACK DOG

ALL BREEDS
WELCOME

Join a support group. There's nothing like being in a
room full of people who understand and share your story.

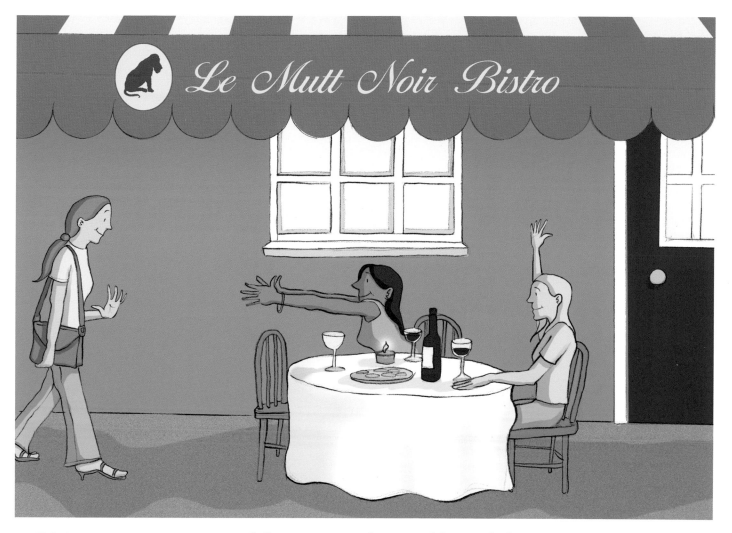

It's important to get out and do your own thing and be with friends. Friends may not be able to solve your problems but they can offer incredible comfort, support and wisdom.

One of the most important aspects of this journey is to constantly remind each other ...

It will pass. It will pass. It will pass.

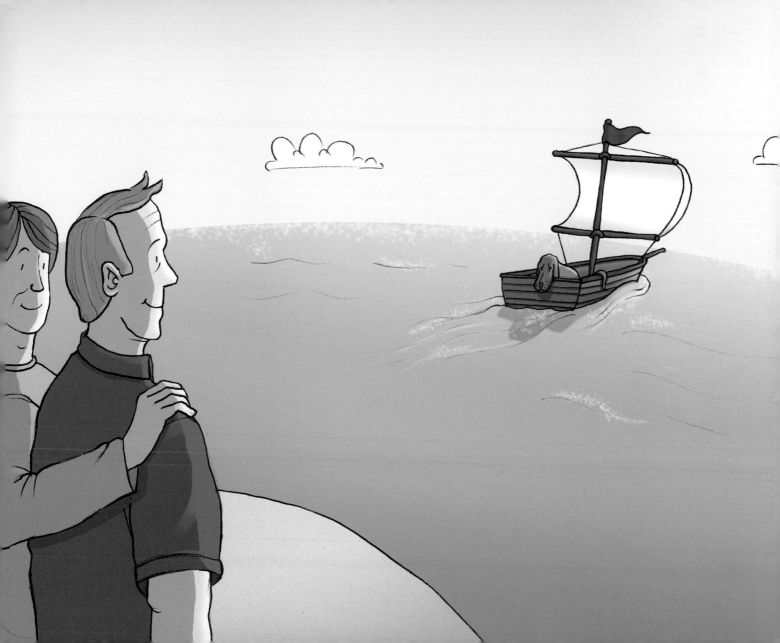

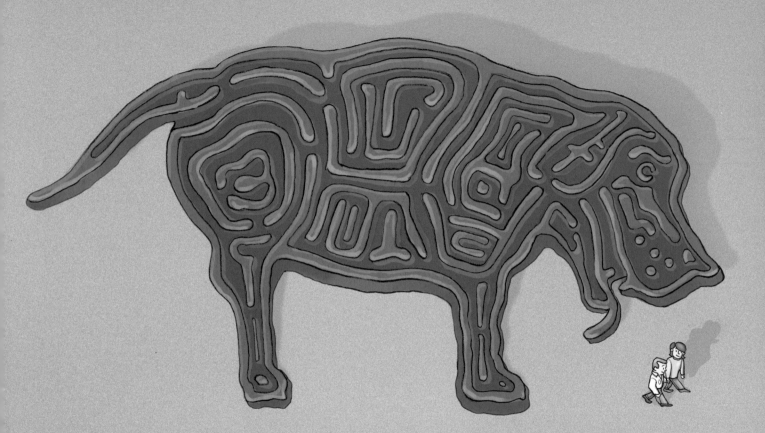

A Black Dog in any relationship can be
confronting, frightening and frustrating but navigated together,
the bond can become deeper, richer and better for it.

'*If life is an uphill slog, imagine the view from the top.*'

Anonymous

BACK-UP PLAN

This is an example of an agreement to act as a safety net for the caregiver and the sufferer as to what should happen if things become difficult.

1) The sufferer should agree to speak up if things are getting difficult. Don't leave it until the last minute.

2) Work out a simple scale for describing how bad it is, from **1** (great) to **10** (very, very bad).

3) Call a trusted friend or family member for help and support.

4) Have an agreement with their doctor that they can be called upon if need be.

5) As a last resort, if you need to go to hospital, know who to call and who to speak to. Know where to go and what will happen if they are admitted.

MENTAL HEALTH PRACTITIONER DEFINITIONS

GENERAL PRACTITIONER:
Also known as the family doctor. They are often the first place to go for help.
They can refer patients to specialists, including psychologists and psychiatrists.

PSYCHIATRIST:
A psychiatrist is a specialist doctor who can diagnose and treat mental disorders,
either with psychotherapy and/or medication.

PSYCHOLOGIST:
A psychologist is a specialist in human behaviour and development. They help people
find ways to function better both emotionally and mentally. Treatment is based on changing
behaviour without medication.

SOCIAL WORKER:
Social workers work with individuals, families, groups, organisations and communities to
address social stressors and provide social support.

COUNSELLOR:
Counsellors are trained in listening and helping people to resolve issues by commonsense
advice and providing problem-solving strategies.

OTHER PLACES TO GO FOR HELP

1) **Doctor** – your GP is your first port of call. (If money is an issue ask your doctor about how to get help that is either free or on a sliding scale.)

2) **Organisations** – such as Depression Alliance, Saneline, MIND, the Samaritans and the BABCP (to name a few) offer vast amounts of quality information and support.

3) **Pharmacies** – have good information on hand.

4) **Natural Therapies** – there are many good, natural, alternative treatments and remedies but these require as much research as the more traditional methods.

5) **Churches, synagogues, mosques, temples and other religious meeting places** – these often have support groups, counsellors or people trained in social welfare.

6) **Universities** – you can often find professional, discounted help in psychology and psychiatry departments and some offer support groups.

7) **Online** – see the following list of links.

8) **Accident and Emergency department of your local hospital** – as a last resort and in a crisis.

SUGGESTED READING

Carter, Rosalyn with Golant, Susan K. (1998) *Helping Someone with Mental Illness*, Three Rivers Press.

Gilbert, Paul (2000) *Overcoming Depression*, Robinson.

Kabat-Zinn, Jon (2004) *Wherever You Go, There You Are: Mindfulness Meditation in Everyday Life*, Piatkus.

Karp, David A.(2002) *Burden of Sympathy: How Families Cope with Mental Illness*, Oxford University Press.

O'Connor, Richard, PhD (1997) *Undoing Depression: What Therapy Doesn't Teach You and Medication Can't Give You*, Berkley Publishing Group.

Parker, Professor Gordon (2004) *Dealing with Depression: A Common Sense Guide to Mood Disorders*, Allen & Unwin.

Sheffield, Anne (2003) *Depression Fallout: The Impact of Depression on Couples and What You Can Do to Preserve the Bond*, HarperCollins.

Styron, William (2001) *Darkness Visible: A Memoir of Madness*, Random House.

Wigney, Tessa, Eyers, Kerrie and Parker, Professor Gordon (2008) *Journeys with the Black Dog*, Allen & Unwin.

Wilson, Paul (1995) *Instant Calm*, Penguin.

Yapko, Michael D., PhD (1998) *Breaking the Patterns of Depression*, Dell Publishing Group.

HELPFUL WEBSITES

www.familyaware.org

www.sada.org.uk

www.mind.org.uk

www.blackdoginstitute.org.au

www.samaritans.org.uk

www.babcp.com

www.undoingdepression.com

www.depressionalliance.org

www.sane.org.uk

www.ihadablackdog.com

From Matthew Johnstone

When I initially handed over *I Had a Black Dog* to my publisher in 2005, I emphatically stated that I didn't wish to become the poster boy for depression; this was part of me, not the sum total. Them fighting words were my way dealing with the pending fear that comes with launching something deeply personal into the public arena. I was also worried that the more you hold on to something the more it will define you.

Creating *I Had a Black Dog*, in many ways has liberated me. Healing wise, it's the best thing I've ever done. It made me publicly confront who I was, what I'd been through, what I'd learnt from it and what I really wanted in life as a result. It has constantly reminded me that I have to walk the talk, to manage my life in a way that keeps the Dog firmly in its kennel. Embracing who we authentically are is one of the best ways of releasing what binds us.

One of the bi-products of creating *I Had a Black Dog*, is that over the last couple of years I've done many talks about coming through the other side of depression to communities, the rural sector and major corporations. This taught me the valuable lesson that helping others helps us to heal ourselves.

No matter the culture in which I was talking, the scenario always seemed to reflect society's attitude towards depression or mental illness. People enter the room, there would be a slight awkward silence, downward stares, the shuffling of bums on seats. After the talk, however, the opposite was always evident; there was a release, the emotional handbrake had been let off and people would **really** talk, often for the first time.

Everyone's life experience is different but when talking about depression, the lyrics of the Black Dog always seem to be the same. And in the same token we may all be different but at the end of the day we all want the same thing; love, connection, understanding and emotional harmony.

One of the questions I was often asked was, 'What advice do you have for the caregiver?'
I'd normally answer, 'You'd have to ask my wife.'
'Well...' they'd say, 'when is she writing her book?'

The truth is we had discussed it but hadn't done anything about it – that is, until Pan approached us.
I was initially hesitant about the project because I didn't think I had another book on the subject in me but one night Ainsley and I sat down and within a few hours we had filled many pieces of paper with ideas and scribbles. **_Living with a Black Dog_** was born.

Ainsley then went out and interviewed many people who had partners, siblings, parents or children who'd been in the company of a Black Dog. Their stories validated much of what we already thought and gave us some truly wonderful insights. For all concerned there was the same sort of watershed that I mentioned earlier.
Most commented that they wished they'd talked like this before.

In this crazy busy life most of us exist in, rarely do we stop and REALLY talk, REALLY listen and REALLY think introspectively. We are all a bit like those water-dwelling insects, who flit around on the surface, rarely dipping below. It's not that we need to constantly talk the 'Deep and Meaningful' but if occasionally we talk with real emotional honesty and intelligence, it can also be incredibly rich, healing and life affirming.

Although this book is by Ainsley and myself I want to dedicate my part of it to her and all the other wonderful people who stand by loved ones with a Dog in their life. It's not easy being with a depressed person but as Ainsley and I have proved to each other time and time again, it can be managed and good can definitely come of bad. We certainly hope this little book helps prove that theory.

Woof woof !!!

Matthew Johnstone

BIG THANKS

Firstly we would like to thank all the people who have supported us in the process of making this book.
Your stories, insights and honesty were inspiring. Thanks to our beautiful daughters, Abby and Luca, for always reminding us what's really important and for keeping our 'chuckle accounts' full.

To our wonderful friends and family for your ears, encouragement, love and support, thank you.

To Professor Gordon Parker and the staff at the Black Dog Institute for their incredible support, advice, friendship and the fantastic work they do in our community.

To Alex Craig at Pan Macmillan, thank you for believing in and supporting these Woof books. Your time, input and friendship are greatly valued. Thanks also to the staff at Pan, without you this book wouldn't exist.

To my agent Pippa Masson and the staff at Curtis Brown who have always been a fantastic support and have helped trot these books out around the world.

To Matthew Cumming for your friendship and helping me build my fabulous website:
www.ihadablackdog.com

To Oil Communications; thank you for all your support and keeping me in employment while doing this book.

To Tanyika Hartge, thank you for helping me out with the finer details of Illustrator.

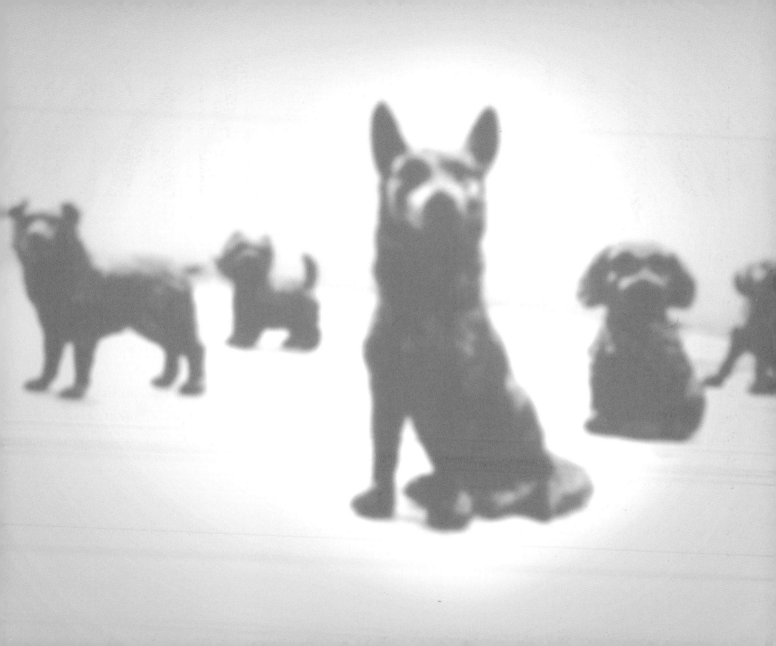